MW01249254

Héarts
GOLD

Hearts of GOLD

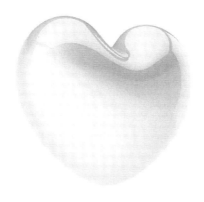

FILEMON LAMAS

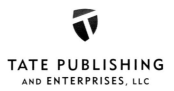

TATE PUBLISHING
AND **ENTERPRISES**, LLC

Published by Tate Publishing & Enterprises, LLC
127 E. Trade Center Terrace | Mustang, Oklahoma 73064 USA
1.888.361.9473 | www.tatepublishing.com

Tate Publishing is committed to excellence in the publishing industry. The company reflects the philosophy established by the founders, based on Psalm 68:11,
"The Lord gave the word and great was the company of those who published it."

Book design copyright © 2013 by Tate Publishing, LLC. All rights reserved.
Cover design by Allen Jomoc
Interior design by Mary Jean Archival

Published in the United States of America

ISBN: 978-1-62510-570-7
1. Health & Fitness / Diseases / Cancer
2. Biography & Autobiography / Personal Memoirs
13.04.19

Contents

Introduction

I am glad that you choose to take this journey down memory lane with me. It will be full of personal experiences and opinions, not to discredit any other beliefs on the subject matter. All these episodes and thoughts are 100 percent true. The story has many emotional ups and downs, and I wrote this not only for the healthy people, but for those who have been diagnosed with diseases that have taken a toll on their families, friends, and themselves. You are not alone in the fight to cure your disease, or cure your loved ones from theirs.

I am going to start off with a personal opinion. I believe people today, like Hernán Cortés, who killed most of the natives in the continent after discovering their precious metals, are very materialistic in many aspects of their lives. Some manipulate or even go as far as killing just to capitalize or to get what they want.

The sad part of this is that they never achieve true happiness in the material items that they fight so hard for. Even after getting what they wanted, most people always end up wanting more. I myself believe that happiness is in the mind, body, and the soul. To be in sync with nature's aura or energy brings peace to those who really want it.

Thanks to La Gran Madre de Naturaleza or Mother Nature, the land provides everything that mankind needs to survive. Knowing that the Earth provides all keeps my heart open to the world and every natural thing in it.

Anyway I have read and studied a little bit about different gods of nature from different beliefs and cultures. I did this so that I could get a better understanding and open my eyes to other points of view of other cultural beliefs. I do believe that there are many natural gods of this world.

I also read and learned about the different tribes of people that used and worshipped all things and emotions of nature. It was pretty vicious and bloody.

What most people never take the time to understand though is that the mighty Mexican Indians made many savage sacrifices. The ancestors believed that if they did not sacrifice to the gods of nature, the gods themselves would grow old and wither away. If this happens they would take with them the harvest, or anything natural that the people used to live on.

The Indians believed that by providing fresh blood and hearts, they could keep the gods young. In return the gods would produce everything in nature that were and always will be the necessities of life.

There are a lot of different opinions and points of view on this subject though. The modern day sacrifices of humanity are less for nature and life than they are for material and capital gains. So which is right and which is wrong?

All the stories are different and all depends on the point of view of the person telling the story.

I thought to myself, *Wow! These ancestors of mine had to go through some very hard struggles than I could ever imagine going through or even endure due to the era and king that was in power at that time.*

There are only ten documented Azteca Kings that I have read about. Either way, I had told myself that if they were strong enough to endure what they went through. Then I would be strong enough to endure what my life has put me through!

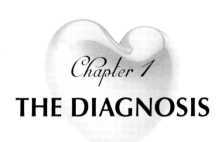

Chapter 1

THE DIAGNOSIS

In 2008, I was diagnosed and has since battled with (AML) acute myelogenous leukemia.

I was only thirty one years old when the doctors and nurses told me I could die if they did not start the chemotherapy treatments right away. The date was May twenty third of two thousand and eight when I was diagnosed with cancer.

I was having massive headaches and my vision was blurring. There were times when it was just pitch black everywhere I looked. I could not see anything during those episodes.

I had gone to the local clinic in Yuba City, CA for the problems that I was having with my pains and sight. The staff there ran me through a CAT scan. They found out that I had two masses growing in the head region of my body. One was in between my brain and eyes, which was shoving my eyeballs forward inside their sockets. That was what created the massive headaches and blurry vision I was having. It was said to be the size of a golf ball.

The other mass was in the right side of my neck.

I left the clinic and walked home in a daze. I arrived still in shock from the news that the clinic shared with me. I sat in a chair in the front yard of my house for about thirty minutes or so when headaches and the vision loss came again.

They were so severe that I lost complete vision in my left eye. My neighbor, who is my friend, saw me in pain and she offered to take me to the local hospital.

Being as stubborn and confused as I was and still in shock from the news, I refused her offer at first. But after about five minutes the pain won and I agreed to let her take me to the local hospital emergency room.

We hopped into her truck and she drove me to the hospital. On our way there, my head still throbbed and I was seeing double. At the hospital, I tried to fill out the emergency room information sheet while I was half blind and in pain. After I finally filled out the form with the right information, I went to sit in the waiting room. It took the staff about fifteen to twenty minutes to call me back to see the doctor.

They then took me to the back and I sat in another small waiting room. This time the wait only took about five minutes. The doctor came in, presented himself as Dr. Roberts with clipboard in hand, and asked a few basic questions, which I answered as best as I could because the pain it was so severe and it was so hard to concentrate or even think straight. I told the doctor about the two masses that they found in the head and neck area that the local clinic found earlier in the day.

He then told me he wanted another CAT scan, so that he could have a better look at the problem. He jotted a few things in his clipboard and then he left the room.

So for the second time that day, I had my head scanned. When they finished the scan, they rolled me into one of the hospital rooms. Dr. Roberts showed up a little while later and told me that I had two masses in my head. I almost wanted to laugh out loud! I reminded him that I had told him that when I first came in. As I sat there he looked at me and asked, "Well, what would you like me to do?" This time I did laugh out loud, head hurting and all.

"I'm the one in pain. You're the doctor, why are you asking me?" I asked him.

I also told him to do whatever he felt was necessary to get me better. He walked away to think for a moment. Then he came back and told me that he was going to have me transferred to a specialist in another hospital in Sacramento. I agreed with his decision and then asked him for something to help with the massive pain I was feeling. He only nodded and walked away.

Two minutes later one of the nurses showed up with liquid heaven in two syringes, which was what it felt like when the throbbing in my head stopped. After sitting for a few minutes the pain was gone and I was able to pass out in the bed.

When I was able to open my eyes, for a minute or two, I found out that one of the paramedics, transporting me to the other hospital in Downtown Sacramento, was talking to me. I could barely understand what he was saying because I was still feeling the effects of the two shots of painkiller that the nurse had injected into my hip. The next time I awoke, I was already in a hospital room. A bit still dazed and confused. I had gotten up and out of the bed because I wanted to take a better look around and outside the door of my hospital room just to see if I could maybe see somebody.

I only had the chance to take about two steps, when one of the nurses popped in through the door. She entered with a smile on her face and began asking if I was okay, or if I needed anything? I told her I was okay and asked her where I was?

She smiled at me and explained that they had brought me from the other hospital to the Neurology section of this one. I guess the doctor had kept his word about sending me to a specialist. The nurse told me that the doctor would be there in the morning. She also said that it would be best if I went ahead and got more rest.

She tried to comfort me ease the nervousness I was feeling from not knowing what to expect. She assured me that the doctors and specialists of the hospital were very good at what they did.

She also said that the hospital had a very high success rate and that I would receive the best help that the hospital could provide.

I thanked her and took her advice to get some rest. I lay down on the bed and a few moments later I was out like a light. Being worn out from all the pain I had felt earlier and the effects of the pain relievers that were injected had caught up with me and only a few thoughts passed through my mind as I drifted off into la la land. It was going to be a pretty heavy sleep. Little did I know the long road of treatments that awaited me.

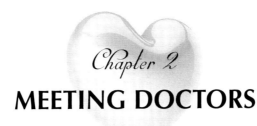

Chapter 2

MEETING DOCTORS

I awoke the next morning, with a nurse bringing in my breakfast tray. She had a smile on her face and greeted me a good morning. She told me to eat up and that the doctor would be in soon.

After I had breakfast and the nurse collected the food tray, three specialists, professionals in their fields of medicine, all came into my room: a neurologist Dr. Rubens, a blood and bone specialist Dr. Carolo, and an eye, ear, nose and throat specialist Dr. Franz. All three presented themselves to me, explaining where they would be participating in the beginning of my hospital stay. They all asked me to sign waivers giving them permission to treat me. This way they could begin with the tests needed to diagnose my illness.

After I signed the waivers, the doctors and the nurses accompanying them left. I was alone and I sat there deep in thought, running through the possibilities of my situation. I was so worried about what the outcome would be or could be. A few hours later the blood and bone specialist

Dr. Carolo came back into my room with the nurses. He was going to perform a bone marrow biopsy on me. So they had me flip over on my stomach. As I watched them lay out the needles that were going to be used for the procedure, the nurses were sterilizing the left hip area of my body and telling me to lay as still as possible. The doctor first began by numbing the outer skin above the left hip bone. It felt like a quick stinging sensation. Then it felt really cold.

Next he went in a little deeper, all the way to the bone and began numbing the outside of the bone area. This was to eliminate any feeling from the penetration of the needle into the bone. He gave it about a minute. Now he was ready to extract the bone marrow. This process felt weird. I felt pressure not pain with the needle he was using. He twisted it over and over, like driving a screw into wood. Like I said though, there was no pain just a lot of pressure on my hip area. In the next step of the biopsy, I felt a pain so sharp, and yet so quick that there was no real way that I could describe it to you in words.

The procedure was successful. He had extracted enough bone marrow to be able to run the test that he needed. They cleaned the area on my body where the procedure was performed and applied a pressure bandage where the needle was inserted. The nurses then instructed me to lie on my back for no less than six hours. This is because there are times when this procedure can cause migraine headaches due to the fluids mixing into the blood stream. Luckily, I didn't have any headaches so I didn't have to go through that kind of pain.

The doctors had me doped up on pain medications due to the tumors in my head. So this was how it went for about three days—I sat in my room, watched television or walk back and forth in the hallways. At times, I would walk just to explore and stop to read the signs on the walls of the hospital. There were also times when I would stop to talk to the nurses.

On the third day after I reentered my room, the eye, ear, nose and throat specialist Dr. Franz came to my room and told me that he was going to perform a procedure on me to have a biopsied sample of the tumor that was in between my brain and my eyes. He told me that he wanted to use anesthesia and put me under in an operating room. While I was to be in this induced sleep, he would shove a steel probe up one of my nostrils to reach the tumor. He would then cut a piece of it off and pull it out for it to be biopsied.

After he left, my thoughts began swarming with every what if questions that ever existed in my lifetime. What if he hits an optical nerve or even worse a brain nerve? I could end up blind or handicapped for the rest of my life. Then to really top it off, Dr. Carolo—the blood and bone specialist—and his nurses came into my room and dropped the "C" bomb in my lap. He looked me over and said you have cancer. I didn't even get the time to recover from all the what-if thoughts I was having about going through the surgery to biopsy the tumor in my head yet. Now, I was receiving even worse news!

Luckily the doctor immediately discussed the steps that we would have to take if I wanted to beat cancer. He wanted to start a very high dose of chemotherapy right away. He told me the sooner the better. Then he turned and walked out of my hospital room with all his nurses following behind him. As he was walking away I could hear him giving orders on how to proceed.

As I sat there with all that was dropped on my lap, the first and only thing I could think of was *wow*! First, it was a steel rod up my nose, probing around in some delicate and necessary nerve endings. Now, on top of that a life threatening disease as well. What was next?

Now imagine. You are laying there in a hospital bed in what is supposed to be the prime of your life. Then imagine the doctors and nurses explaining to you that because of the disease you were just diagnosed with, a common household cold or fever could cost you your life in a matter of an hour. It was nerve-racking experience to my system. Never in my life did I ever imagine that I would be going through such trials in health and medicine, especially, not all this at the same time.

I mean what was I supposed to do? If I denied any of the treatments I could die. *Wow!* There were not many pretty pictures being painted for me. Yet, because of the lessons life had taught me up to this point. I think that I handled it about as well as anyone could have. I tried to be positive considering all I had been told in less than three hours time, so all I could do was hope for the best. My thoughts just kept flying through my mind and I could not concentrate on one thing. The only thought that actually stuck was that this was not happening. Not to me. Yet, no matter how many times I thought it.,it did not change anything. It was happening to me and faster than I had ever experienced in my life. There truly was not much I could do about it other than roll with the punches that life was throwing at me. With all the ups and downs, it felt as if I was on one huge emotional rollercoaster and that there was no end to it and whether I liked it or not there was no getting off it or slowing it down.

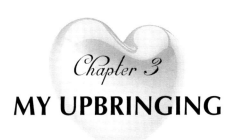

Chapter 3

MY UPBRINGING

After receiving all the bad news from the hospital staff, my mother came into my room. She had gotten the news from the doctors and nurses in the hallway before coming in. Now if not for my Mexican culture upbringing, where the men in the family must be strong for the women and children, then I probably would have broken down and filled my bed sheets with enough tears to float a boat in. She was there though, so I had to stay strong. Plus if I had broken down and cried she would have felt it worse than I did.

I could only imagine what it felt like to watch your child or children be diagnosed with a disease that you had no control over. The only thing you can really do is hope for the best and let fate decide if your time in this world has come to an end or not. Nobody can escape fate. I don't care who you are or who you believe yourself to be. Only nature has the power to control our outcome, without human intervention, and outlast us all.

My mother was always a very strong and proud woman. She was born and raised in McCallen, Texas. Her circumstances in her life made her grow up at a very young age. She told me that she lost her parents in a car accident while she was still a teenager. The accident also left a younger sister in a coma at the hospital. When she came out of it, my mother was the one who explained to her younger sister how their parents died. As they grew up, the sisters helped raise and support each other as best as they could.

During my childhood, my mother cared for my three sisters and me as best as she could, considering the limited resources that she had available to her. She raised us in a small town, but the good thing was we never needed anything.

You see, my mother had a real big heart. She helped the hungry, and those who are cold as best she could. Those that she helped, after finding work would repay her kindness with freshly picked fruits and vegetables and whatever else my mother needed.

Due to her kindness a lot of *jente*, or people admired and respected *mi familia*. I was lucky enough to sit with a lot of the older Mexicans that came from Mexico to work where ever they could find it. They would sit outside with my family and me around a table in our front yard. We would sit there almost every night listening to them sharing their stories, legends, and the politics of all the different states in Mexico. Since I had no older brothers, the men that came to share their stories would always treat me like I'm their younger brother. I would sit outside and wait for them to get home from work, and I always wonder what kind of stories they would tell that night. This was something that I found a lot of pleasure in.

You see, the Mexicanos have a lot of legends of the devil, witches and witchcraft, and animals. Sometimes, their stories are just a bunch of trying experiences in their lifetime just like a poker game, which could turn into a Wild West situation because nobody liked to lose. Some would even bet their whole paycheck, and then remember that they couldn't afford it after all.

So life was pretty exciting in my childhood. I would absorb like a sponge all that they told me and what I witnessed, and take it all to heart. For us, it's an honor to be proud of our culture, which has struggled through many generational gaps, and injustices done to us by different people and beliefs as we try to seek a better life for ourselves or our families.

All cultures have a similarity of pains, feelings, and sometimes a little too much pride, which can sometimes get us into a lot of trouble. Either way I was glad to be given that opportunity to listen to these stories. I have always used a lot of the *consejos* or advice that one gains from listening to other people's hard life's lessons. I have a habit of saying that you will never know. But these experiences could happen to you down the road and knowing the outcome of someone else's similar experience could save you a life time of regrets or pain. At least that's the way I see it.

There are many times that history repeats itself. It is always better to have a heads up on some of those situations. The lessons and morals have a way of repeating themselves. Same situations, different people, and if you're open minded enough, you may be able to catch it, and prevent the same mistakes or from happening again.

Chapter 4

COMING OF MIRACLES

All the patients that came through the hospital were treated with almost everything that they could ever ask for. The nursing staff was always helpful and concerned about all the patients and their recovery while under their supervision. A lot of the times, they would go out of their way to make patients and their families feel more comfortable while going through their hardships. If not for these doctors, nurses, social workers and other hospital staff, I probably would not be here to tell you my story.

At this time, I found myself with no income and no food. My mother had only Social Security, and with this she had to pay her bills and rent. So her resources were very limited as well. Yet, my mother did everything that she could to make me feel like everything was going to be just fine. My sisters also helped me with what they could afford financially. They did not like to see me going through such a hard trial in life. So I also had to keep in mind that they had their lives to live and children to feed.

I started feeling like the world was closing in around me. You see, the doctors and nurses had told me that I had to move to the city, so that I could be closer to the hospital and treatment centers. I lived like three cities away and with no income; I felt like I did not know what they wanted from me! I just could not afford it! Plus it was not much of a choice. I had to afford it or die due to the treatments. If my hair had not already fallen out by then, I would have been pulling it out by the bunches.

There was a light at the end of all the darkness and misery. It came to me in the form of friends and people who cared about me and my health. I had been raised around and had gone through so many negative environments, that it was what I was used to. I have seen so many people lie, steal, and die. They kill each other for drugs, woman, and even over a point of view. It was sad that I had gotten used to the negativity, hate, and selfishness. I had forgotten that there are still some people out there in all the chaos with true hearts of gold like the Indians from Aztlan. These included the the American Cancer Society, and Leukemia, Lymphoma Society and all the social workers that took the time to find all the resources available to me and my family in our time of need.

These selfless organizations and people who came together with the funds to help me be nearer to the hospital and treatment centers where I would be receiving my transfusion, infusions, and any other antibiotics or my system's blood counts should they need to be replenished. These were the days when all of the stresses and worries came into my life. These were also the days that the induction stage of my chemotherapy treatments began.

I was also relocated to the (BMT) Bone marrow transplant unit from the Neurology part of the hospital. This was after they diagnosed me with the cancer and started the strong doses of chemotherapy treatments. The tumors in my head began to shrink, which meant there would be no steel rod probing up my nose or anywhere near my brain. That part was a huge relief to me. That was really not something that I would like to leave to chance even if the doctor was a specialist. That was a big whew!

All these trials in life really teach you how good you have it and yet so many people take it for granted. There is always something in life that can always be everything you want it to be. Do you know that if people spent more time of their lives looking at making positive changes instead of complaining about the smaller things, they might actually be able to have a genuine smile on their faces? Too much time wasted looking backwards means that you are always going to have more mistakes than you would actually want. It would be best to pay attention to where you are going instead of where you have been. You can get a lot farther in life that way. Even I had to work on that one myself.

To get to where you want to be instead of where you have to be is freedom in itself, and the only way to that is to set your goals and achieve them. Do not allow everyone else's drama to blind your choices in life, unless it affects you personally. You can struggle a lifetime trying to fit into what people would want you to be, but you have to stop and ask yourself: Is this really what I want to be? If not then you are going to have a harder time struggling with yourself and your decisions and living miserably.

It's too much effort instead of just being you. Trying to satisfy everyone else would be like living with a split personality disorder, where you deal with your emotions and everyone else's opinion. The thing to remember is that you have a choice to do something about your life. You can make it harder and complain about how nothing changes or change what is hard in your life. In the end you're either in control or you're to blame for not taking control of your life. There is really no one else to blame except you. By accepting this, you give yourself the power to be happy.

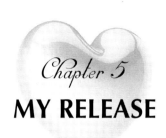

Chapter 5

MY RELEASE

It was during these very stressful days that I felt like I was walking around everywhere in a heavy daze. I felt like I did not have control over anything. For me, it was like the worst feeling in the world. It did not even matter if I had been a bodybuilder or just your average Joe. I felt weak in my body something that I wasn't used to. Plus, I had to find a place to live or stay with the minimal of funds that I had available to me. My world was collapsing around me and I was helpless to do anything about it. I believe that I was in severe shock due to my ailment.

The reason I said this was, it was around this time that I had the opportunity to meet Ted Summers one of the few wonderful social workers that had been assigned to my case. I was so stressed out that I could hear everything that he was saying to me, but for some reason I could not comprehend any of it. He tried to explain to me that the situation was not as hopeless as I felt it was. He tried to point out and explain all the resources that he was able to tap into so that I had somewhere to stay in the city near the hospital and the Infusion center.

Like I said though, I was in shock and really didn't comprehend any of the information that he was trying to explain to me. When we finished talking we shook hands, he gave me his card and let me know that if I had any questions not to be afraid to ask him about it. I shook my head answering yes. This was just to get away and to sit alone for awhile. It was something that I felt I really needed to do at this time. Since I really did not understand anything he was trying to tell me anyway, I just kept getting more frustrated with myself for being so weak in body and mind.

After a month and a half, the day finally came when they released me from the hospital. To be honest, I was ready to go anywhere that wasn't a hospital room. After being released from the induction cycle of my chemotherapy, thanks to all the staff and the social workers, I had somewhere to stay in Sacramento. I now had three days to report to the Sharing Place, where all the beautiful cancer organizations, helped pay for my stay. The agreement though was that if I didn't show up before the appointed time to register for the room, I would lose the spot that they had saved for me. There were also a lot of other families, who needed the assistance as well.

You know even to this day, there are more and more families having someone that they love being diagnosed with cancer and other life-threatening diseases, where the hospitals end up being overcrowded, and these families and patients have to stay at other locations less convenient for them. Then it really becomes hard for patients, doctors, and all the organizations that help fund and give care to the families in need. Any donation that people can spare to these organizations is more than appreciated by me and other families that may find themselves in my situation or worse. There are always fundraisers located everywhere. So please don't be afraid to participate if you ever come across one. Even, just your physical support is good enough to show your support to the cause to save lives.

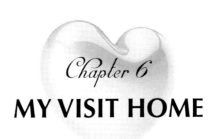

Chapter 6

MY VISIT HOME

The first stop was at the Sharing Place so that I could check in and reserve the time in three days to come back and occupy the room. After doing this, we were ready to go home so that I could visit my family that could have been maybe for the very last time. I really did not know how everything was going to turn out. Especially with how the doctor and nurses had explained to me how simple it could be for me to lose my life.

My third oldest sister Rebecca had come all the way from Utah, so that she could have her bone marrow tested and maybe be my donor. You see, sometimes they have better luck matching when it's a sibling with the same parents compared to different mothers and fathers. So if she did match my DNA, she was willing to donate her bone marrow for me. So we went back to the hospital, and the staff did all that they needed to do so they could run the test needed. When she had finished giving her sample, she drove us to a supermarket so that we could stock up on the foods and necessities that we needed for our stay at the Sharing Place.

After pulling into the parking lot and finding a spot to park, I had to sit in the car while they did all the grocery shopping because my chemotherapy treatments already eliminated my whole immune system. This left my body in a neutropenic state, which meant, that I had no immune system—not even to fight off someone's allergies. A simple sneeze or a cough could have been enough to pass on a cold or fever that everybody else's body could fight off, but to me it could cost me my life. I wasn't going to take that chance even if I did have on a mask. There was too much risk and the price was death just for a walk in a crowded area. If someone coughed into their hand, grabbed a door handle or railing of some sort, the chance that I would get sick was anywhere from seventy to eighty percent. So I sat there waiting for them to come back from inside the store. I was lost in my own thoughts when they finally came out and loaded the groceries into the car and headed home to Yuba City so that we could finally relax. When we pulled into the drive way, I let out a sigh of relief to finally be back home. Later we sat outside talking, making up for lost time, and catching up on each other's lives.

After a while, I looked down the street and decided to visit Ronald the man, whom I worked for before I was diagnosed with leukemia. He and his family are also among the people whom I consider as having hearts of gold and

I could never thanked them enough for the support they gave me and my family during our time of crisis.

So I got up from where I was seated, told my family that I would be right back, and took off walking to where he lived. He was at home and we talked. I told him about my diagnosis, and all the worries and concerns that I was going through, and the problems I was facing.

He listened while I poured my heart out to him. After I was done, he told me that he too had been diagnosed with leukemia. The difference between our diagnoses was that he was told that his cancer was terminal. He said that they had told him that he was not going to make it. Yet he did!

I believe fate and destiny brought me to meet this man and his family in my lifetime. He made it clear that I need not worry about where I was to live in Sacramento. He said his son owned property, an apartment, in the downtown area, which wasn't far from the hospital where I was to go and had to be on a daily basis for needed lab work and treatments. He also made it clear to me that he would cover the deposit on the apartment that I was going to move into.

After hearing all this I felt that my heart broke that I wanted to cry and I struggled to control my emotions because never in my life, had I been able to meet so many righteous and caring people.

I'm really not used to allowing people to help me without being able to give or do something in return. That would be the Mexican pride in me—that as a man I will never bow my head in shame or beg people for food but I'm always willing to work for it instead. Yet at this time I found myself in a position where I really did not have those options.

Anyway, he was able to relieve some of the stress that I had on my mind. I thanked him and walked back home to share the good news with my family.

I walked up the driveway with a bigger smile than when I left them and shared with them the good news. They seemed to be a little relieved about the situation we found ourselves in. Even though they did not show it, I knew that the worries that weighed heavily on my heart and mind, weighed heavily on all of theirs as well. So I tried to make everybody feel a little better by cracking jokes so they could keep smiling instead of being all stressed out.

Since I was the one going through everything, I know I could not control the way things would turn out. But I really need not be around sadness or it would have broken me down in every way possible. My body already felt weak from all the induction of chemotherapy and I still had so much more to go through.

This was only the beginning of my long journey that I was to live through. So I had to keep my mind, body, and emotions as strong and positive as I possibly could. It was the only thing that I had left that I truly had control over.

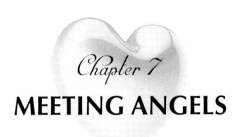

Chapter 7

MEETING ANGELS

After spending the three days with my family, which I felt was not long enough for me to truly enjoy them under the circumstances, it was time to finally go back to the Sharing Place. Now it was time to get back to the treatments at the hospital and infusion centers.

Upon arriving at the Sharing Place, I had to ring the doorbell. This was for the security of the patients and their families staying there. Bob, the manager opened the front door and invited my mother and I in. We followed him into an office where he explained the house rules for our stay at the Sharing Place. I then filled out some forms. After I was done, the manager gave us a tour of the house where he showed us all the areas that were accessible everybody. He then led us to the room where we would be staying, handed us the key, wished us his best, and went about his normal everyday duties.

The room had two beds, a bathroom, and a swamp cooler because during the summer it gets pretty hot in these areas. The Sharing Place also had two family rooms with television, magazines, and bookcases with many books to choose from. It had a small courtyard connected to the buildings that you could access through two doors made of glass. One of the glass doors lead back into a family dining area. This was where all the families staying in the house were able to eat their meals together. This and the kitchen area were the only places that food was allowed to be.

The kitchen area consisted of three large refrigerators, two stoves tops, three ovens, two sinks, dining ware and utensils, which were plates, silverware, and drinking glasses. They also have some food and bread that were donated for families like mine that did not have much. Since we did not have much and what little we did have, we had to use sparingly.

One of the amazing facts about the Sharing Place was that everything in it was donated by many caring people, businesses, and other families that were doing pretty good for themselves and wanted to share their wealth.

After finally settling in and putting everything away, I had to make it for an appointment at the Infusion Center. This was to be on a daily basis, so I was told. So we would go through the hospital that was in the entry way of the Sharing Place. This was where we could catch a shuttle bus that ran back and forth between both hospitals. One hospital is for women and children, the other for everyone else. We waited there, talking to some of the other nurses that worked in that hospital until the bus showed up. Then on we went. Luckily it was a free service provided by the hospitals for doctors, nurses, and patients. This was good for me considering that I was low on funds to begin with. It would drive and drop us off in front of the main hospital that was right next door to the infusion center, which was pretty convenient for me at the time.

The infusion center was on the sixth floor of the hospital. I would check in and be given a chair to sit on and a pump for the infusions themselves. While at the center I would have my blood drawn for lab work and would receive whatever my body needed infused through the pump into my body.

I would also stop to talk to the new social worker Tisha Jones that they had assigned to my case. I would share with her all my thoughts and worries and she would research and find everything that she could find that she felt I would need to make my life a little easier while going through this very traumatic time of my life.

Once again the kindness and unselfishness of these people opened my heart, mind, and soul. By this time my mother and nephew had switched places on who would stay and watch over me, so that they could help me with whatever I needed because the chemotherapy had done a number not only on my immune system but on my body as well.

We were also running low on the food and money that we needed for the necessities that we had to come up with for our stay. The stay at the Sharing Place cost twenty dollars a night. I also learned that the American Cancer Society had already depleted the funds that they donated for my stay, which is understandable, considering the increasing number of people being diagnosed with cancer each year. I would find it difficult to find money in a downed economy. Yet these organizations worked so hard to find more revenue to be able to help people like me, who had fallen on hard times and could not pay for their treatments let alone their stay while undergoing these treatments. There really was no choice! The only other option was death. I do not think many people would even have to stop and think about it twice.

Now it was during this visit at the Infusion Center that I was approached by Richard, a man whose wife Karen was also a patient in the BMT unit of the hospital during the induction of my chemotherapy. She had fallen and had been sitting on the floor for about fifteen minutes. So while I was routinely walking my rounds in the hallway to exercise my legs instead of just laying on the bed. I had happened to look in her general direction and caught a glimpse of her sitting on the floor. I thought it very odd to have this older lady in her condition to be sitting on that cold and hard hospital floor. So while walking past the nurses station I brought it to their attention that the lady was sitting on the cold floor. They all got frantic and rushed into her room to aid her back into her bed. They wanted to make sure that she was all right. They discovered that she had fallen trying to stand up, so after they got her back in her bed and made sure she was fine, they left her room.

Not too long after I entered and also wanted to make sure that she was all right. After introducing myself, Karen thanked me and we talked for a while about our disease and treatments. The conversation then had lead to how long we had been in the hospital for this stage of our treatment. She told me that she had already been there for five months nonstop. I told her that I had barely started, so I only had a month and a half under my belt and was already going stir crazy. We ended the conversation by joking that she had me beat by three months. We got a good laugh out of that one for a minute.

Anyway, her husband approached me in the hallways of the Infusion Center. He said hello and asked if I would follow him into one of the empty hallways of the wing we were on. He had started by explaining to me that he and his wife had overheard my social worker and I talking about my situation and my issues.

He apologized for being so intrusive into my personal matters. I told him not to worry about it there really wasn't anything to hide. He then said that after listening to my issues, he and his wife had come to the decision to lend me a helping hand. He took the time to explain to me that he and his wife were doing well for themselves and at that time handed me an envelope, which contained two hundred and forty dollars.

Once again I found myself struggling with my emotions. I had a sharp pain in my heart and tears welled in my eyes. It was to me such a gesture of generosity coming from a couple that I had only known for a day. Yet, hearing my story and the stress it was bringing into my life, these two wonderful people with hearts of gold came into my life.

I am very fortunate to have been given this opportunity that fate had laid out for my life at this time. These people and their act of kindness will always be held deep in my heart, no matter where we may find ourselves. I will always remember them and by doing so I will always find a smile in my life just knowing that there are still people out there that care not only for themselves but for others as well.

After thanking him and giving him a big hug, my nephew and I headed to the park in front of the hospital to wait for the shuttle bus to transport us back to the Sharing Place. My Nephew had accompanied me during these treatments to hold me and make sure that I didn't fall down or hit the floor especially since there were days when my body was so weak from the treatments that I would feel like passing out even from the simple motion of sitting down or standing up. My nephew would be there to help me during those episodes.

But since we were already near a grocery store, we decided to pick up a few items and food that we would need. Of course entering the store in my condition was a risk in itself. I had to use a facial mask over my nose and mouth just in case someone had sneezed or coughed, or after doing one or the other touched an item in the store. With my immune system completely gone that time, catching a cold or having a fever would be fatal.

So I cautiously entered the store and allowed my nephew to touch and bag all of the grocery items that we purchased. We then headed to the park in front of the hospital and sat on the grass waiting for the shuttle bus that would transport staff and patients back and forth between both hospitals and the Sharing Place.

The shuttle bus was very convenient for us especially in the condition I was in. Imagine if there was no vehicle to transport us to the hospital and Sharing Place; with what little funds we've got, we might end up taking that five to ten mile walk to get to both destinations. In my condition, that walk could have been the death of me!

Luckily there wasn't as many commuters on the shuttle bus as there were on a regular transit. This was less risk to me and my health, which for me was more like a flying carpet ride because I didn't have to walk on pins and needles worrying of contracting a cold or fever amid a crowded transit. Again, my system during these days was what doctors and nurses called neutropenic, which meant I didn't have any immune system to defend me from those simple contaminators.

As I was thinking about all this, the shuttle bus emerged from one of the corners of the hospital grounds. With all the shuttle drivers knowing us pretty well being their regular commuters, the shuttle then departed as we settled in our seats. The shuttle driver Mario then looked at me and smiled, and said that this was the last ride in the direction of the other hospital where I was staying. He said that after he would drop us off, he then be transporting staff members from the hospital to the light rail station. He was referring to those staff members that commuted using the trains.

I thank the driver and was relieved that we had caught the shuttle ride in time to get back to the Sharing place.

You see the shuttle and public transit were my only options to get back and forth from all my appointments. Without funding for a vehicle or taxi on regular basis I felt like I was playing Russian roulette with my life. There was, however, an only as needed resource provided by the hospital, that the social worker had found for me. They would give me a voucher for a cab if the timing on my treatments ran later than the schedule of the shuttle or on my weekend appointments when there's no shuttle service, which wasn't easy for me considering that my Infusion Center appointments were and had to be on a daily basis— seven days a week. Yet, somehow we were always able to make it and there were times just barely.

When we finally reached our destination, we said our goodbyes to the driver and unloaded our bags. With bags in hand, we had to walk the rest of the way to the facility. As always the commute back and forth from my appointments would wear me down so that every time we reached the facility during these treatments, I would go directly to my room and lay down, depleted in every way possible. I had very little energy and strength through out the whole process of my chemotherapy treatments. My nephew would either pass out in the other bed, or go watch television in one of the family rooms. As for me that night, I went to bed and slept.

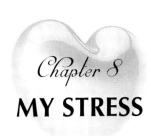

Chapter 8

MY STRESS

The induction process of my treatments was complete and all the infusion visits to the center had raised my blood levels to a safe and restorative functioning level. This meant that my body's bone marrow had begun to produce stem cells again for itself enough to keep the blood levels from falling and climbing at very slow but steady pace.

It was at this point that the doctor decided to continue with the next cycle in the chemotherapy treatments. He explained that it would be series of about four cycles and then the bone marrow transplant itself. All I could think about was how unfair I thought it was that as soon as my system had started recovering, he would decide to knock me through a loop with another dose of chemotherapy. This always meant that the weaknesses and all the risks would start all over again.

What else could I say? No? That I didn't want to go through the treatments? Are you kidding! With my life hanging in the balance between life and death, choosing to at least go through this process gave me a fighting chance. So it really did not matter I had to endure everything that was thrown at me. Each cycle consisted of me being hospitalized for at least a week. The dosages were a very potent mix of chemotherapy in two bags every other day. So it was pumped into me within six days. I would then be released to the Sharing Place and start the daily infusion center visits all over again. So that I could be infused with the glucose that was needed for my body to have the chemical buildup that keeps us alive and healthy.

During this cycle in the hospital, I met Mike a young man about my age that was afflicted also with AML. We both had the same doctor and treatments to go through. The only difference was that he was one cycle ahead of me in his treatments. We met while I was thinking and trying to plan for after the cycle. You remember that I said that everything that was given to me was on a limited budget. I was thinking about how my resources and funds for the Sharing place were running low. I was afraid that after they were exhausted, they would not be able to provide housing for me. I was worried that if I did not have the funds to stay there, would they have to kick me out? So these troubling thoughts filled my mind. The more the staff told me not worry the more frustrated I became. I found myself pacing the halls of the BMT unit with these thoughts running over and over through my mind.

He noticed my walking back and forth with a troubled look on my face. He approached me when I turned around from the lap that I had just taken in the hall. He extended his hand to me and introduced himself. We shook hands and I also introduced myself. Mike then asked me, why I looked so troubled? He also made me laugh when he said that the faces I was making while I was lost in thought were pretty funny looking. I told him that I had not even noticed I was making faces until he had mentioned it to me. We then burst out laughing.

He asked me what my diagnosis was and how far along in the process was I in. I told him that I had been diagnosed with AML and was in my first cycle after the induction. After hearing this he took the time to explain some of the procedures that I had to look forward to. He also said that the procedures themselves weren't all that bad, and that the best thing we could do was to try and stay as positive as possible. This would make going through everything a whole lot easier. In all honesty, it really did.

During our conversation he took the time to explain some of his worries and concerns to me. This time it was my turn to lend him an ear. He told me that he served in the military for a few years and after coming home was diagnosed with the disease. That for me felt unfair, that fate would take away so much from one person with his responsibilities after having gone through so much. It made me realize that there are many families out there that are going through their own battles and struggles dealing with it in their own ways. So after realizing that I wasn't the only one suffering from the disease, and after hearing the man's story, I was able to let go of some of the pent-up pressure that I felt.

I thanked him for helping to put my mind at ease and wished him the best in all his future treatments. He thanked me and wished me the same. I then returned to my room with a clearer mind than before as I continued to think about my situation.

The next issue I had to consider was where I was to live. Since the doctor and nurses told me that I had to move nearer to the Sacramento hospital and the resources at the Sharing place were nearly depleted, I began to worry again because I barely had any money in my pocket and I had nowhere else to go. You can just imagine the stress and pressure that I began to feel again.

I began to feel unsure of what or how I was to accomplish anything that I had to do. I felt like there's a deep, deep helplessness overwhelming my being and there was no escape from it. What made it worse was that everything was happening so fast that my mind went on the fritz. I could not concentrate to make decisions. I felt as if I was exposed to the world like a newborn baby who could not care for itself.

By this time my mother had returned to watch over me. I noticed that she would excuse herself to go out for a lot of walks. I believed that some of those walks were made so that she could go off somewhere and cry and avoid trying not to upset me. I then realized that she was just as stressed out if not more stressed out than I was. Think about it. She was watching me and I felt that she also felt that there was so much to do and so little time to do it in. She also had to keep in mind that her baby boy was close to death and that the whole time she had to try to remain strong for me. That would have to take its toll on anyone and I love her for that. I also felt her pain as well as my own.

And so I maintained my composure as best as I could. I really did not want to stress her out anymore than she already was and cause her a heart attack. With so much going on around us and everything that was coming to me was so fast that I once again fell into a shock-like state of mind. My mind was not registering some of the information that the staff were trying to give me. It was so complicated for me that in the end I had no choice but to leave everything up to fate about what was to happen first—the money running out at the Sharing Place or being able to get the money to move. This was the hardest thing that I had to admit to myself at the time and one of the hardest decisions that I ever had to make in my life. I'm so **bull**-headed sometimes that this truth was eating me up from the inside, but I couldn't do anything about it but just lay there on the bed.

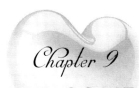

Chapter 9

MY FEAR COME TRUE

A fter going through and completing the cycle of chemotherapy. I was released and it was planned for me to continue on to my daily infusion center visits. My skin had dried out, I had lost a lot of weight, and I was getting a lot of dizzy spells. It was during these times that my mother would always assure me that everything would turn out all right. She would try to comfort me by telling me that everything would fall into place. Even though I was full of worries before she would even talk to me, I found comfort in just her words and had faith in everything that she would tell me.

I lay there in that hospital room, which could turn out to be my death bed if caught a fever, being neutropenic—or having no immune system at all. So believe me when I tell you that any caring words shared with you by your family is something that anyone would find comfort in.

The next morning it was time again to have my lab work done at the infusion center. After they drew what was needed from my PICC line or peripherally inserted central catheter line to be tested and sent to the lab.

One of the IV (intravenous) nurses was cleaning the dressing over my PICC line. This is the tube that ran directly into the main vein up my left arm. This is a procedure that had to be performed on a weekly basis. If the temperature was hot outside and the area collected sweat. Then the dressing had to be changed as well. This was due to the risk of infection. After receiving the results and being cleared to leave the infusion center I returned to the Sharing Place. While there, I went to the kitchen to make something to eat. I was standing there making myself a couple of ham and cheese sandwiches when the new family that had come to stay at the Sharing Place entered the kitchen. I was then introduced to the bravest eleven-year-old boy I had ever met. Danny had been diagnosed with a tumor in his head like I had been. It had been discovered that it was a cancerous one located behind his left eye. The difference between his cancer and mine was that his cancer had been put into remission once before and it had returned.

As we made our lunches, Danny discussed about all the procedures that the doctor had planned for him and his treatment. He seemed very positive in his attitude and outlook of what he was facing. I sat and listened to him and his parents as they explained to me the previous procedures that he had been through. This was when he shared something that made my heart sink. It made me realize that what I was facing didn't seem that bad in place of his and what he had to look forward to. He said that this time they were going to have to remove his left eye! It was hard to believe that someone so young could sit and explain the procedure that the doctors had decided to perform on him. Yet, there he was with his warrior spirit and brave heart. He and all his glory, with a smile had inspired me to be more positive. I thought to myself about all the obstacles that he could face in life and at his school with all the children that could ridicule him. There are a lot of children that like to blurt out many hurtful things just to show off and not really care about what the other person has had to endure. Or at least they did that when I was a kid. So I thanked him and his parents for sharing their story with me and wished them well throughout all his future treatments. I truly hoped that all would turn out well for them.

I carried my food to the table and while sitting down thought to myself what a brave kid he was. So I sat there and ate while looking out the window, enjoying the view of the flowers and trees, and thinking about my future treatments. As I finished my sandwiches and cleaned up my mess, I headed outside to enjoy a cigarette with my mother. We headed out the door out into the parking lot talking about what was to come. I sat on a curb and lit up my smoke.

As we were sitting there talking, a man approached us as asked for directions. He began sharing with us that he had a two–year-old daughter who had been diagnosed with leukemia as well. He had been working all day in the fields and had driven hard for over fifty miles to be with his child knowing that his child had been diagnosed with a life threatening disease like cancer. Everyday must have been harder and harder on him with nothing else to think about on his drive but his family and ill child.

As we were about fifteen minutes into the conversation, I started to sweat heavily followed by cold shivers and light-headedness. I did not know what was going on with me. So I got up slowly, and let my mother know that I was going to go inside and lay down. I hoped that I could relax and that it would pass. But as I took three steps across the parking lot I began to lose my balance and the next thing I remember was lying on the asphalt of the parking lot looking up at the sun beating down on my face. As I lay there I watched two birds above me flying in circles like buzzards over my corpse. I became very frustrated with myself for being so weak and not being able to lift myself up and walk. Feeling this weakness irritated me very much. So I gathered my strength and stood up a second time. Boom! Down I went again! This time when I came to, I was being held down by my mother and the man that we were talking with.

By this time someone had alerted the emergency staff from the hospital for women and children of whose parking lot we were in. The only thing I could hear was my mother and the man asking me not to try and get up again. I was still pretty disoriented from passing out and falling on the asphalt. The emergency staff had finally reached me, lifted me up, and put me into a wheelchair.

They secured me and rushed me through the emergency doors of the hospital and immediately began connecting the IV drip lines with a saline solution to rehydrate me. The next thing I knew the staff was cutting away all my clothing off my body. It was then that I was asking myself if I had died for a minute? All my bodily functions had shut down, releasing urine and fecal matter. In other words I had pissed and crapped on myself. I felt very embarrassed laying there in that hospital bed having other people cleaning me up. I did not like the feeling of weakness and most of all not being able to care for myself. Even while this was going on, I also had to give the information of my doctors and treatments. You never knew what medicines could counteract with a system so vulnerable that it might cause death. So they jotted down the information, and called Dr. Carolo, informing him of my situation. It took about a half hour or so to stabilize me and allow the ambulance drivers to transport me over to the other hospital and back into the BMT unit.

They ran a series of test to determine the cause of what could have triggered such a reaction from my body. After the results of the analysis had come back to their desks, it was apparent that the cause was a skin infection that had entered into my system through the PICC line in my left arm. Somehow a piece of dead tissue had entered the incision and caused all that to my body within a few hours. So Dr. Carolo prescribed for me to receive antibiotics through my PICC line. I was to be released after everything was secure and back to normal, or at least what normal could be considering my treatments. After that, I was to continue my daily routine of infusion center visits.

It was a pretty scary episode that I had experienced that day. I had been taken down by an infection that I could not see and there was nothing I could do about it except try and survive it. To be completely honest I was very unsure of how the results of my future treatments would be. I mean to see how truly weak my body had become scared me that I could not defend myself physically or other than leaving my life in the hands of Dr. Carolo and his nurses.

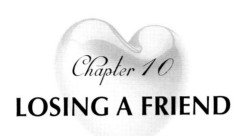

Chapter 10

LOSING A FRIEND

It was during this stay in the hospital that I was going over what the doctors and nurses had told me. In the beginning they shared with me about how any small cold, fever, or infection could kill me. I thought to myself, wow! They really weren't kidding! While I sat in my room, reading the newspaper about all the problems going on in the world. I came across an article that caught my attention. It was an article about Mike, the man I had meet during my induction phase. He was the same age as I was and shared his story with me during my time of need. He passed away from a cold or fever leaving behind a beautiful wife, and his two young children. I said to myself she must be a very strong woman to go through such a challenge in life and still be able to put together a memorial service in memory of her husband. My heart went out to them.

I left my room to walk and think about the article I had just read in the paper. After about a lap or two, I stopped at the nurses station to share with them what I had read. They also expressed their sadness for the man's family.

The time finally came when my body had recovered the best it would and Dr. Carolo had decided to release me to go home. At this time, I got word that my friend, Ronald the man I was working for before I was diagnosed with cancer, kept his word and sent me a check for the deposit on the apartment with his best wishes that everything would go well for me during all my treatments.

While going through all these phases in my treatments, there were many times that I find myself neutropenic or having no immune system to fight off colds, fevers, or infections and it is a constant worry for my health as shown by the previous chapters.

I was finally able to move into my new apartment, but it had no furniture or beds. So my mother and I had to sleep on the floor. We ended up having to sleep on the floor for a couple of weeks. Going back and forth to the hospital to make it to my appointments was a challenge in itself because I found myself neutropenic and was risking catching illnesses especially since all I had was public transportation.

The local bus stops would run close enough to the hospital that I could be dropped off and I would walk it most of the way. The other challenge was walking the rest of the way to my destinations. You see walking for me was difficult due to light-headedness, a feeling like your going to pass out every time you stood up.

It was during some of these walks in between the bus stop and hospital that I would have to stop every so often to throw up on the side of the road. I found myself feeling sorry for the people who lived along the street that led to the hospital. You know having to wake up to see me puking my guts out and sometimes in there front lawns. I would like to apologize to those people, I am truly sorry for that.

I however made it to my appointments every time though, so that was a good thing. After getting there I would have to sit in the chair, have my blood work drawn up, sent to the labs, and wait for the results. This time the results came back that all my glucose counts were high. The doctor after receiving the results came to the decision that it was time to begin the second cycle of chemotherapy. So off I was again another long week into the hospital for another stay.

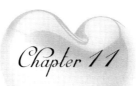

Chapter 11

THE COUPLE OF HOPE

A s I walked that day to the catch the bus, I sat there thinking to myself, how I had made it this far through out all the treatments and life's struggles that I had been through. Everyday I would look into the mirror after getting out of the shower and see a thirty-one-year- old man, who at the time had no control over life or death. I had to accept that as the truth, and make the best out of it. I tried and always smiled about the choices that I had to go through regardless of what would happen. Live or die it was in the hands of my creator and the medical staff that worked for the hospital that I was on my way to. The bus was coming around the corner now so I had to stand up and let the dizzy spell pass.

If I didn't, I probably would have fallen on my face just trying to climb up the three steps that led into the bus. After climbing into the bus and paying the toll. I went to find my seat. The good thing was that I meet a lot of interesting people on the bus.

This day I meet a young girl who was a paralegal running errand for her law firm. We sat and talked during the ride. She told me that she was also taking classes to learn the Japanese language. She wanted to move to Japan and teach the children there. I told myself that would be kind of cool to be able to move to different countries and see the differences in cultures.

After listening to her story, I explained what I was going through in my treatments. She sat and listened to my story with sadness on her face. When I had finished my story, describing step by step what I had been through, she looked at me and apologized. I told her there was no reason for her to apologize to me because it wasn't her doing this thing that I'm going through in these trying times of my life. So, I smiled to reassure her that everything was fine. She smiled back and by this time the bus was reaching my destination. We then said our goodbyes and I wished her luck in all her schooling and legal research. She smiled and wished me luck too. So I left the bus with my mind back on making it to the hospital for admission to start my second cycle of chemotherapy. I walked the five or so blocks it took me to get there. Before reaching the front doors I ran into one of the shuttle drivers that used to transport me back and forth from each hospital when I was staying at the Sharing Place. We had a quick conversation about how we had been doing, but being pressed for time and having to check into the hospital, I had to excuse myself and wished him the best. I turned away while saying goodbye and entered the hospital through the revolving doors that was located in the front of the hospital building.

After entering I approached the receptionist desk and immediately began joking with her about how I wanted the biggest suite that they had and that the money was no object and be sure not to forget the room service. Also that no wake up call would be needed, because I was sleeping in! She immediately began laughing. She thought that was the most hilarious statement coming from a cancer patient with more things to worry about other than the obvious. It would always help me to be more positive about what I was going through by giving away free smiles to those that looked like they needed one.

There would be many times when I would talk with people who would always find themselves complaining about the smaller things in life and in the middle of the conversation would stop and take a look at me all bald and thin from the chemotherapy treatments that would kill all good and bad blood cells alike and everything else in your body. They would then stop and think about themselves; how they did not really have it that, bad you know? They could have been going through what I was going through.

Anyway, after signing in, I found out that they already had a room ready in the (BMT) unit for me. I thanked the receptionist and she led me to the elevators to reach the unit. After reaching the unit, I immediately started cracking jokes with the nursing staff telling them the reason I kept coming back was because I missed the food! They sat there and laughed with me for a minute. I then went to my designated room and got settled in. After folding my clothes and putting away my cosmetics, I began my walks up and down the hallway to see which patients were new. I came across Val, this petite woman who had a look like she was carrying a mass of weight on her shoulders. I walked up to her and introduced myself and we began to talk.

I started by listening to her since she looked like she needed an ear to release some of that weight she was carrying around. Val told me that she and her husband Denis were schoolteachers and that he had been diagnosed with cancer and was in one of the other hospital rooms down the hall. She looked really stressed out about what could happen with her husband's health. I sat there and looked at her, I felt sorry that she felt kind of like I did. You know the feeling? It feels like you have no control of the outcome of life and death. Her issue was that she had no control over the health or outcome of her loved one. So I sat there, shared my story with her as well as my point of view about everything that was going on with me. I understood where she was coming from, but I didn't like to see her suffering for something that she couldn't change or have any control over.

I explained to her my point of view on how spiritual enlightenment could help her through her trying times in life. Val agreed with me after hearing what I had explained. She then told me that after Denis's diagnosis, they had started to seek other forms of enlightenment in place of religion, but had a hard time achieving it. I told her that the reason it was so hard for them was that they cannot control everything in life. There are some things that you just have to let take their courses. The only thing that you can do is help it along by having more positive experiences for yourselves.

Put a picture in your mind about what this means: Imagine life on a leaf, floating on a river of emotions, if you don't lean this way or that way then you will never know how or what you're going to feel on your journey in life.

You can however guide your emotions somewhat to hit all the rapids or calmer currents of the emotional river that we ride on. Even though you cannot control it all, you can still enjoy the ride. Or you can keep flipping over your leaf with all the negativity and life feels like it gets harder and harder where it feels more uncontrollable. Then you have to work twice as hard just to get back on your leaf. You must know how to get your emotions back in control. Val thanked me after our conversation, and left telling me that she wanted to go for a walk and think over all that we had talked about.

She returned about thirty minutes later and asking me if I were all right, and if I needed anything. I told her I was all right and thanked her for her concern. I then asked her, how Denis was coming along. She told me he was doing well considering the treatments, asked me if I would like to meet him? I agreed and we left my hospital room for her husband's room down the hall.

Upon entering she introduced us. We said our hellos and began discussing each others treatments. After talking with this couple for awhile let me tell you, these two people belonged together. I thought they were so funny arguing back and forth over the smallest things. But I knew it was out of love for each other that they did it, so I sat and laughed as they where talking and explaining to me their jobs, livelihood, and concerns going through their minds. All I could do to ease their worries was to explain my experiences in some of the treatments that they had to look forward to.

We finished talking and I was feeling kind of tired. So I told them I would visit them later and went back to my room to lay down for awhile. When I got into my room, one of the nurses was already hanging a bag of chemotherapy. After being connected to the hoses of the pump, I sat and thought of how I was being pumped full of this poison that was going to save my life and at the same time sucking the life out of me.

I finished my second cycle of chemotherapy and was released to go home to recover and allow my system to recuperate. I was also instructed to visit infusion center the next morning. So I got home lay down and got some much-needed rest without the tubes hanging out of my arm.

The next morning I showed up at my infusion center appointment and sat again with the social worker Tisha Jones, since I was still having money issues and we were still trying to figure out the best way to take care of my necessities. We came up with one way to save money, by going to the public transit office and applying for a discount due to my handicapped status. So Tisha got me the form that I needed to get this accomplished. As I was leaving her office, I ran into Denis and Val again. Upon seeing each other we both lit up with smiles. They told me they were happy to run into me again, because they had been talking to each other and decided to give me a gift. They then handed me a prepaid gift card for a hundred dollars.

Once again in my time of need, the chance meeting of two more unselfish people with hearts of gold came to my aid. They also smiled and asked me if there was anything that I needed for my new apartment. I told them that I needed a bed for my caregiver and if they had it a space heater. Their faces lit up with huge smiles and told me that I was in luck and that they had both and would bring them for me. They said that one of their mothers passed away and left them with a lot of stuff from her estate. I gave them both a hug and thanked them for being there for me. They said it was no problem and it actually made them happy that someone could put the stuff to use.

When I left the infusion center once again I went to the grocery store to pick up the necessities and food that we needed. Once again the challenge of entering and exiting the grocery store without catching a cold or fever was constantly on my mind. It was also very difficult to walk around the store without vomiting all over the place because all the chemotherapy had me feeling nauseated most of the time. You see from all the chemicals flowing through my body it made my stomach weak and at times it made it hard to eat. Dr. Carolo told me that during this process if I had the urge to eat anything, then I should do it. With chemotherapy in your system it kills your urge to eat normally. Honestly, it was pretty hard to keep a good appetite while going through my treatments with my stomach full of toxins. He always told me that I should drink as much fluids as I could drink to flush all the chemicals out of my systems. That was one of the things that nearly drove me mad while I was in the hospital. I was always having to measure the urine put out from my system. This means that I just could not go to the bathroom because I had to measure and document this every time I used the restroom. The nurses and doctors had to keep numbers of the amounts my body put out to make sure that it was extracting the poisons that was saving my life and not endangering my safety. So if I liked it or not, it was absolutely necessary. I had to make sure my body was doing its duty. If my body was not functioning like it should, then they would have to turn up the saline drip and flush it manually. They would have to give me laxatives and all that good stuff that forces the body to function when it does not want to. So my drinking as much fluids as I possibly could was in my benefit.

There were many days when I would just pick at the food that was served to me and I would have to force myself to eat. Anyway, it was one of those very trying times and standing in a grocery story was just one of the many.

While standing in the line waiting to pay for my purchases I would talk about all the local businesses and the money they were making due to the hospitals in the area. After paying, it was off to the bus stop with all my goodies. Getting them home was a job in itself. I was lucky enough to accomplish it every time though, so I was grateful for that much. While waiting for the next cycle, I had to go in to receive a spinal tap. This I had to do every time I had a cycle of chemotherapy to go through. This was to check the fluids and blood cells that the marrow in my spine was producing. So I went to my appointment and received a spinal tap. So after you get a spinal tap you are supposed to lie on your back for about eight hours or so. So that's what I did sitting at home waiting for the next cycle.

Chapter 12

PAINFUL MEMORIES

As I was nearing my third cycle of chemotherapy, I fell ill with spinal fluid infection. I did not know it at the time, but I couldn't even stand up without doubling over with pain shooting through out my body. It was so painful that I would have to stop whatever I was doing, and then a tingling painful sensation would run up my legs and into my spine and continue on into my shoulders.

It would then creep up my neck and all the way into my head. My body would lock up on me and I would begin sweating so bad drops of sweat would fall from my face on to the front of my shirt. It was so much that it would leave my shirt sticking to front of my body. Yet, due to how stubborn I was, I went through these pains for three days, every time I stood up. So when I finally built up the courage to call it in to the hospital. The nurses told me to come in a soon as possible and get checked out. So I went ahead and scheduled to go into the infusion center in the morning. I was feeling very nervous about how to get on the bus in my condition. Weak and in pain, with all the sweating, oh, I was just so miserable. One of the reasons it took me so long to call the hospital was that I was stubbornly hoping that it would go away since I had no cold or fever just pain. I would think to myself, that as long as I did not have the first two symptoms, I might be able to sleep it off. If my system were normal it might have worked, we will never know. When I went to bed that night, I closed my eyes and hoped that the morning would bring with it less pain in my body. I was wrong. The morning came and when I pulled back my blankets to get out of the bed and get ready for my appointment. The pain came even harder, but I had no choice. The longer I sat there, the worse it would get for me. So I got up showered and dressed taking about an hour or so due to the pain doubling me over. It was so bad the only way I could feel any relief was to lay back down in my bed and wait for it to subside. Every time I would get back up, I could not even take five or more steps without doubling over and sweating on myself. I almost wanted to cancel the appointment to the hospital, because I wasn't sure if I was going to make it. But just knowing that if I did not go to the appointment the pain would continue to be there and get worse was enough for me to grit my teeth, do what I had to do in the house and make it out to the bus stop to wait for the buses to arrive.

After reaching the benches at the bus stop, I was so queasy from the pain that I felt like I was going to throw up. As I sat there trying to control this urge, the bus came around the corner and I did not know if I was going to make it. As the doors opened, I approached the driver paid my fare and asked him to use his garbage can for the ride. He looked at me kind of funny not sure what to think. I explained to him my treatments and what I was feeling. So now he understood a little more how I felt and agreed to let me use it as I sat in my seat hugging the garbage can for all it was worth.

He began driving towards the downtown hospital while I shook and sweated for the ride until we reached the stop I was getting off at. As I exited the bus, I thought about the five city blocks I had to walk to get to the Infusion Center. At the time they felt like miles in my condition. I lowered my head and just kept putting one foot in front of the other until reaching my destination. I was so relieved when I finally made it there. To this day I really do not remember looking around, just focusing on my feet to get me where I needed to be. I entered the building and stood before the elevator that seemed like forever when the doors finally opened letting me in. I pushed the button to reach the floor where the infusion center was located. After exiting the elevator, I stumbled around the corner and as soon as I entered the sight of the nurses. They took one look at me—standing there, full of sweat, trembling from all the weakness I felt—and rushed me to one of the chairs and immediately got me started on fluids and antibiotics that would help my body control its system a bit more. This way they could investigate the cause of the reaction my body was putting out. They kept asking me questions, but in the misery that my body felt at the time. I was honestly not in the mood to answer any of them. After sitting for a minute, I passed out in the chair due to the relief the fluids and antibiotics had brought to my system.

The staff figured that I would probably be there for a while recovering, so they decided to send me across the hall into the doctors' offices and placed me in one of the examination rooms. As I sat in that room, I had a very caring nurse Patti, that sat and watched over me for the next two or three hours. I sat there in that chair passed out while she did crossword puzzles and checking on me. After those two or three hours, I was then stabilized enough to be transferred over to the BMT unit of the hospital. So Patti left the room and returned a few minutes later pushing a wheelchair. She asked me to climb in and off we went. As she pushed me through the halls, I was feeling a whole lot better and so being the man I am. I could not help myself and started cracking off jokes the whole way to the BMT unit. I told Patti that was pushing me in the wheelchair that she had forgot to use her blinker when we had come around the corner. If she wasn't hanging onto the chair she probably would have fallen over I had her laughing so hard. I finished up with how I would take the chair into the shop and have it painted with racing stripes on the side and a Daniel Boone raccoon hat on top of an antenna attached to the back. This is how it was all the way until I had reached my hospital room.

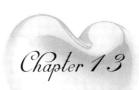

Chapter 13

MY REOCCURENCE OF FEAR

Since I was used to all the procedures that I had been through, while in the BMT unit, I now had it down to a science. There were many times during my stay in these kinds of facilities that if you do not keep your mind busy you can literally go stir crazy. One of my favorite things to occupy my time was go into the family room and raid the freezer for the different flavors of popsicles and ice creams that the cafeteria of the hospital was kindly providing for all the patients and families that stayed in the BMT unit of the hospital. They were so good that I would do this about every three hours or so. As always while on my walks up and down the hallways, I would stop at the nurses station to joke with the staff there about how I had been through so many procedures that I had them down and if that qualified me to be a nurse to. They would laugh with me and explain to me how I needed to go to school for all the lessons and procedures that nurses must learn to conduct their everyday jobs.

While I was standing there joking at one time, the results of one of the lab works had come back. They read the results and called Dr. Carolo, who decided I needed a platelet transfusion, because they were kind of low. Without your platelets your blood would not clot up to stop you from bleeding if you were to get a scratch or a cut. So they rushed to pick up what they needed and sent me to my room to lay down and wait for the transfusion. When the nurse Corrin returned, she had hooked me up to a full bag of saline solution and was giving me some Tylenol and Benadryl to counter any reaction that my body would have to the transfusion pushing blood back into my veins. About fifteen minutes after starting the transfusion, I started breaking out in an uncontrollable itch all over my body. When I looked down at my arms, they both had broken out in goose bump-like rash all over my body. Corrin the nurse that was documenting the transfusions date and time with everything else that was given to me was standing next to me when she noticed me itching all over the place and told me that she would contact Dr. Carolo right away to see what he would like to happen next to stop the reaction.

As she walked out of my room, I turned to watch television and that moment was all I last recalled. As I came to, I was hearing the voices of the staff yelling my name out to me over and over. I noticed that I was now wearing an oxygen mask that had been placed over my nose and mouth area. There was also about a half dozen nurses swarming around my bedside. They were the ones yelling my name to me until I came back to my senses and was able to reply in return. It was then that I had realized that it had happened again! My body had shut completely down to a bad reaction. My system had quit functioning for a minute. I had crapped and urinated all over myself while vomiting. My head had a pretty good-sized knot on it as well. My guess was when my body had shut down; I had fallen sideways and had hit my head on the railing of my hospital bed.

In all honesty, while this was happening I really didn't feel anything at all. The nurses kept asking me even after I had responded to them if I was all right. I kept trying to assure them that I was. After they were satisfied that I was up and running again, they told me that I had scared the shit out of them! I then asked them how they thought I had felt! First breaking out in all those bumps then coming too with all the nurses circling me like a bunch of buzzards! I was scared too! They said yep, he's back to his self. So they monitored me closely and got my blood levels back to somewhat safe blood levels. The antibiotics had taken care of the infection and the time had come that I was well enough again to be released and go home. The plan was for me to sit at home while going to infusion center visits for lab work and await my third cycle of chemotherapy. So there I waited as patiently as possible for what destiny had in store for me. I could not do anything to change my fate except try and enjoy what little I had and be as happy as possible while doing it. That's pretty much all we truly have in this lifetime of ours. You never realize it though until you actually go through something so life threatening and changing that you or no man has control over it—no choice but the hands of fate.

Chapter 14

GOOD NEWS, BAD NEWS

While I was waiting for the go ahead on my third cycle of the chemotherapy treatments at my apartment. I received a phone call, from my mother. She called to tell that she had gone to a local clinic in Yuba City, her area and had received some bad news. She said that she too had been diagnosed with cancer—breast cancer.

She told me that they were hoping that performing the surgery would remove the cancer and for her to begin her treatments to this disease, so they could prevent its spread, just in case they could not remove it at all. So now, not only was I going through these treatments due to this disease, but now it was infecting my mother too.

So we sat talking on the phone for a long while discussing about staying positive and doing our best to overcome anything that we had to go through to successfully survive this disease. We neared the end of our conversation; we talked about the easiest ways to avoid getting infections in our PICC lines that the hospitals had placed in our veins.

Luckily, my Mother was looking at everything in a positive way and assured me everything would be okay. So I also tried to have a positive outlook on everything was to come for both my Mother and I. I was so proud to have such a strong woman for a Mother.

I made a few visits to the Infusion Center and talked with the staff and social workers about all the treatments that my mother and I had to look forward to. They gave as much advice as they could to help ease the stress and worries in my mind. It was just there were so many things going on in my life that I had no control over and had to learn to just accept it.

Then Dr. Carolo decided it was time to start my third cycle of chemotherapy. Well, I decided I was as ready as I was going to be. The next day I once again got up, showered, dressed, and went out to the bus stop to wait for the trip to the hospital. I had everything I needed for the week's stay during the cycle. I had even taken some of my dirty laundry with me to save a little money. Saving even a little bit was very helpful in my financial needs.

So I got dropped off and went walking to the hospital. After walking through the doors I went to the receptionist desk and signed in. They had me wait in the lobby until the BMT unit called down for me. It seemed that there was a vacancy, but the room had to be sterilized first, before I could occupy it. After a few moments' wait, they finally called to have me come up into the room.

Since I was considered a veteran in the treatments I was going through and I was a couple cycles ahead than most of the other patients, I would try to meet the new patients, talk with them about how the treatments felt, what to expect, and what made things easier for me. I truly believe that I was able to put many of their minds at ease as what was once done for me when the shoe was on the other foot. I would also share some of the stories of the other patients that I had met while going through all the treatments. Then as always, being the comedian that I am, I would end up telling a couple of jokes and leaving everyone with smiles.

While I was sitting being pumped with one of six bags of chemotherapy that was scheduled for this cycle, Dr. Carolo came in and talk to me. He told me that he was happy about how I had been doing while going through all my procedures and he wanted to move the bone marrow transplant ahead of time.

After hearing this information I thought to myself: *What no fourth cycle. Whooo hooo!* He also explained that he would be able to use my bone marrow and that it should be healthy enough to do the transplant with. He told me that using an unrelated donor could have up to thirty five percent chance of death as compared to five percent if you use your own bone marrow. I joked with him that it would be like playing Russian roulette. Yet deep inside of me, I thought, *holy cow that was a huge gap in between percentages of death*, especially when it's my life that we are gambling with.

So you can imagine the relief that I felt lifted off my shoulders after Dr. Carolo chose the procedure with less risks involved. After explaining the different types of transplants and risks, he also explained the next steps that we would be taking to prepare for the transplant itself.

The first step was to, of course, wait for my body to raise the blood count at a safe enough level for me to be dosed twice with a very high and very potent chemotherapy. This procedure was to clear out any residual infected cells from my body and my bones. After a little time of recovery from these two doses.

The next step was to go over to the main Infusion Center in the next building. This was to harvest and collect stem cells that were newly released by my bone marrow. He said that it was a process that would more likely take anywhere from five or more days.

After they drew my blood and sent it to the labs to check the count, which was for the specific fact to ensure the count of my blood cells was high enough in my body to be collected. Now whether if I did or did not have a high enough blood count, I was still to be injected with a chemical called Neupogen. This chemical forces your bone marrow to produce more stem cells into your bloodstream. This would cause the bones in my body to ache as if they were growing. That would just have to be something I would have to take the pain medication for and do my best to deal with the pain. After that they would collect the amount of good and healthy, clean stem cells.

Then it would be time for the next step. The next step would then be the bone marrow transplant itself.

After hearing all these procedures that he had planned for me to go through, I told myself: *Well, this is something I have to go through to save my life*. So I looked over to Dr. Carolo and then said, *okay. Let's do it*. Then I flashed him a smile of hope.

I was really very scared and worried about the outcome of everything that I was to look forward to. It was more the not knowing what these procedures would feel like. I figured that after everything else I had been through, I was hoping that it would not be that bad. So I took a deep breath and hoped for the best. What else could I do?

Chapter 15

HARVESTING OF MY CELLS

While sitting with Dr. Carolo, he had also told me that before going in to start with the stem cell collection, I would have to set up an appointment with a radiologist to insert a catheter into the main vein, which would allow them to collect and flush straight from the source of my lifeline. So I called and made the appointment on the next spot available for me to come in and have the surgery completed. Next, I showed up at the doctor's office where this procedure was to take place. They had me fill out all the necessary consent forms that they needed to continue with the procedure. After filling out the paperwork, I had to change into a hospital gown so that they had better access to sterilize the area where to the tube was to be inserted especially since they wanted to insert the catheter tube into a vital and very dangerous artery of my body.

Remember an infection could kill me if any germs or bacteria where to come off my clothes and into the area of the insertion. So I changed into the gown and laid in the examination room. As I sat there awaiting the doctor to come in and perform his procedure, Amanda, the nurse had entered and began explaining what I was going to be put through. She reached up and lowered the upper half of my gown and began sterilizing the area where the catheter was to be inserted. She asked me if I was comfortable. I was very nervous and answered that it really did not matter because I had to go through it regardless. If I did not go through with it, it could literally cost me my life. She smiled at me and told me, "Yeah, but you still have a choice to go through it or not." I smiled back and said, "Let's do it."

I really did not have a choice. I mean, life or death, which would you choose? So the doctor entered, presented himself as Dr. Douglas, and took the time to professionally explain how he would go about performing what he had in mind. I lay there while he pulled out a syringe and explained to me that this was to numb the area where he would insert the tube. So Dr. Douglas inserted the needle, massaging the area around the injection. This was to spread the medicine and kill the sensation in the area of my chest that he had marked to insert the catheter. I felt a bee-like stinging for about fifteen seconds or so. He pulled out the syringe and gave it about a minute to take affect.

Dr. Douglas reached over and grabbed a blade of some sort using it to make an incision in the chest area and began by pushing the tube little by little into my skin and into my artery. I could not feel it completely, but what I did feel was a whole lot of pressure from his hand inserting the tube of the catheter. The tube itself was about the width of a number two writing pencil, and about six to twelve inches in length. He took his time performing this procedure so the sensation of the pressure lasted for a while. As I was lying there in that bed listening to Dr. Douglas and Amanda having a simple conversation of their everyday lives, it had come to me that these people where so used to what they were doing that to them it seemed like nothing was going on out of the ordinary. Yet, it was my very first time that anyone had ever performed this kind of surgery on me. It made me feel very nervous in as weak of a condition that I found myself in, sitting there watching the doctor shove a tube into one of my main arteries.

He finally finished what he was doing and asked Amanda to clean up around the area where the incision was made. When I looked down and saw the catheter itself, it had three ports sticking off of one tube. This was for all the injections, extractions of chemical or bloods could be made through. She asked me to lie still as she sterilized then stitched up the skin around the tube. When Amanda had finished, she smiled at me and asked how I was feeling. I answered that I was feeling as okay as any cancer patient would feel after all the treatments. All this with a smile on my face. She said that I was free to leave when I was ready.

So I left heading back downtown to my apartment to sit and await the stem cell collection. The area where the

Dr. Douglas had made the incision began aching with a pulsating sensation, letting me know that the numbing medicine had worn off. This pain continued for a full twenty-four hours.

So now at this time I found myself sitting in my apartment with my caregiver Terri, who was kind enough to sit and listen to me as I rattle on about my worries. I would like to send a special thanks to her and her family. She too has a heart of gold and I'm glad to have been able to meet her. To my caregiver: "Thank you for taking the time for being there for me when I most needed you."

I sat there with her nervous from not knowing what to expect once I reached the Infusion Center. These thoughts were the most troubling for me during the days that I was awaiting for the stem cells to be collected for the bone marrow transplant. I sat there hours on end thinking, until I just came to the conclusion that I could do nothing more than to accept it. No matter what were to happen, it was something that I had to go through to save my life, so there was really no other option other than death.

When the day finally came for my first appointment, I was becoming overwhelmed with nervousness and insecurities not knowing what to expect. So we got ready, went down to the bus stop, and waited for the bus that would drop us off to the area nearest to our destination. After walking the rest of the way to the Infusion Center, we sat outside waiting for the front doors to open. So we sat there enjoying the beautiful water fountain near the entrance way of the Infusion Center building. You know I found peace in looking at something so beautiful instead of worrying about what the unknown was that awaited me inside the building.

After about thirteen minutes, the security guard approached the doors and unlocked them. I took a deep breath, stood up, and entered the building. As we entered, we walked over to where the elevators were located and stood before the elevator doors and waited for them to reach our floor and open. When they finally did, I thought to myself how time seems to slow down when you're playing with your life in other people's hands. It was one of the weirdest feelings that I have ever experienced in my life.

To better explain it, it felt like one minute was like an hour. We reached the waiting area of the Infusion Center and sat waiting for the nurses to arrive. It felt like an eternity but in reality it was only five minutes.

We saw the nurses Betty and Cherri, who seemed to be in good spirits, approach us. As always they assured me that it was not going to be that bad. That all it would be was just like sitting in a chair hooked up to the machine through a hose that would be connected to the catheter that was between my neck and upper chest.

Well, it seemed a lifetime ago since the catheter procedure but now I'm here in a room in the Infusion Center going through the stem cell collection process, sitting here in a room with the three ports hanging out of my chest, connected directly to my lifeline. Betty approached and told me that she first had to draw a blood sample to send to the labs for a glucose count. She drew blood from one of my ports. After collecting a blood sample, she would flush the line that she had used with a liquid called Heparin. This was an every time process after using one of the ports to prevent clotting of the tube and infections.

I sat there in the chair for about an hour waiting for the results. It was time. The results were back from the labs. Betty approached me, chart in hand, and shared with me that my bone marrow had not produced a sufficient amount of stem cells to begin the harvesting of cells. They looked at me with smiles on their faces and asked the next question: "In which one did I want two in?" I said huh? They laughed and reminded me of the Neupogen shots I was to receive so that my bone marrow could produce more stem cells for the next day.

So I smiled and joked with them about how I knew that their real intention was to harvest blood for the vampires that ran the hospital—as many pints of blood that they were collecting from all the patients on a regular basis.

So while they were giving me my injections they were also laughing their heads off. They had given me three shots, two in one arm and one in the other. The medicine that was in these syringes was so thick, you could feel it burn as it entered the muscle tissue. After giving me the injections, they sent me home with both of my arms pretty sore.

I left the Infusion Center for the day and waited at the bus stop for the bus to arrive. My caregiver Terri and I sat and talked about how everything was going with my procedures. The bus arrived and we headed home. When I reached the apartment, I lay down, watched television, and tried to relax. I, however, ended up thinking about what I had already gone through, as well as how my Mother was going through her treatments. I realized how this disease takes its toll on the body and mind, how it just slows you down. It makes you put everything in perspective and if you're healthy enough, to be grateful to be given a second chance in life to be a better person. With all these thoughts in my head, I turned off the television, closed my eyes, and fell asleep waiting for what the next day had in store for me.

The next morning I woke up, jumped into the shower, got dressed, went down to the bus stop, and rode the bus to the Infusion Center. It was pretty much the same routine. I showed up at the infusion center doors at seven thirty am. The Nurses Betty and Cherri showed up, we shared pleasantries and they unlocked the doors so we could go in. I would then sit in the chair, had my blood drawn so that it could be sent to the labs for the glucose count. They flushed the line that was used to draw the blood, and told to wait for the results.

So I got up out of the chair and raided the snacks and drinks that the infusion center provided for all its patients. I sat down with all my goodies and took the time to use the restroom. I washed my hands thoroughly, turned off the light and went to sit back in the chair. On each individual chair they had a small television, with headphones that you were able to use during your infusions or procedures. So I put it to use while we waited. About twenty minutes or so later, the results came back from the labs. My body had just barely produced enough stem cells to begin the collection. After reading the charts, the nurses Betty and Cherri called it in to Dr. Carolo, who then gave them the go ahead to proceed with the harvest. They came back to my chair, gave me the news and began hooking up the tubes to my catheter.

They went through the checklist to assure that everything was properly connected before turning on the machine. I sat there watching as my blood got sucked out of my body, filtered, then separated into two bags. The rest of my blood got circulated back into my body. It was pretty crazy, once you watch it getting put into action. The whole process was kind of fascinating. While I was sitting there getting filtered I really did not feel any change, I felt okay. This process took about five hours.

They had collected what they could for the day and unhooked the tubing from my three ports. They also took the time to flush each individual tube out. Now, I had to sit and wait for Dr. Carolo's decision, if I was to come in the next morning for more stem cell collection.

Dr. Carolo decided that I was to come in and be put back in the chair the next day. After a little bantering with the nurses, they again gave me three shots of Neupogen. After the injections they sent me home. The only thing about going through this procedure and all the injections is that you do feel a little lightheaded. So feeling this way, Terri my caregiver helped me all the way to the bus stop. She made sure that I did not lose my balance and made it safely to my apartment. After riding the bus home, Terri helped me up the stairs and into my apartment so that I could lie down, get some rest, and recuperate from all I had been through for the day. I lay there for a little while when finally the lightheadedness went away. So for the next five days that's how the process went for me—back and forth to the Infusion Center for the collection of stem cells. The reason for the five days was to make sure that they had collected enough stem cells for the transplant itself.

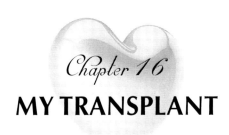

Chapter 16

MY TRANSPLANT

The next step was to prepare for the bone marrow transplant itself. When I spoke to Dr. Carolo, he told me that I was to be in the hospital for this procedure. The first step was that I was to be dosed twice with a high mixture of chemotherapy. After receiving both doses, I would be given two days to recover. Then it would be time to go through the transplant.

Then, I was to stay in the hospital until my blood levels and my systems came back to safe enough level for me to be released. This was to be pretty similar to the induction stage of my treatments. When all the treatments began, I was full of worries and concerns about how I was going to survive all the treatments that I knew nothing about. Now I had been through it all and was coming to the major transplant itself. *Wow!* Well, I guess after everything was said and done, I was ready for it.

The day finally came when I was to admit myself into the hospital so the process could begin. That day I hopped on the bus and walked the rest of the way to the hospital. The whole time I was thinking to myself how I was hoping that all would go well. At the hospital, I had myself processed and led upstairs to my room.

The procedure began right away as soon as I had put my things away and settled in. The first treatment and dose was to consist of sixteen bags of one kind of chemotherapy. So I sat for about two days going through all these bags. About halfway through the treatments my stomach began to feel toxic. It was so bad I could hardly keep the little food I could eat down.

So after two more days of letting me recover from the first round of the treatment, the next round began. This consisted of two bags of a different mixture of chemotherapy. Having so much chemotherapy running through my veins and body, made me feel so toxic that I was surprised I was not glowing in the dark from all the radioactive chemicals. I was waiting to see a whole bunch of radioactive signs pop up all over me. So after finishing both doses, they gave my body and system a little bit of time to recover.

Then it was time for the transplant itself. When Doctor Carolo and nurses came into my room, I was very nervous not knowing what to expect is what made me feel this way. The nurses Gina and Mandy began to set up the equipment that was going to be used. While they were busy doing this, Dr. Carolo was explaining how the procedure was going to work. He seemed almost as excited as I was from everything that was going on around me. He told me that ten frozen bags would be thawed out in lukewarm water. These ten bags contained the frozen stem cells that they had collected from me at the Infusion Center. They would then hang each bag one by one upon a hook and allow nature to take its course.

What this meant was that gravity would pull the stem cells from the bag into the IV tube and flow slowly into my body. If it where to pump into me too fast, it could cause me to go into a shock. So now they were ready to begin. Gina and Mandy came to me and handed me a bag of hard candies. They explained to me that during the procedure it would make it easier for my throat if I were to suck on the candy while being infused with the cells.

I was pretty confused at that time and I did not understand what they were talking about. As soon as the first bag was hung I figured out that they knew exactly what they were talking about. As soon as the stem cells hit my blood stream, I felt a very strong choking sensation overcome me. It came to a point where I felt like coughing and choking at the same time. Gina and Mandy were right though the hard candy did make it a lot easier. The whole process took about an hour.

After we finished, Gina and Mandy picked up and removed the equipment from my room. It was time for me to play the waiting game once again. My blood levels were down, but climbing back up steadily. There were a couple of other patients that were either going through the chemotherapy treatments or the transplant as well. Those patients that had gone through the transplant were having as much trouble eating as I also did. The problems of eating and drinking lasted about ten days.

Please believe me when I tell you that this part of the recovery was not that fun at all. Even with my sore throat I was still harassing and joking with the nursing staff on a regular basis. I had to stay busy somehow. The only thing that did anything to soothe my sore throat was drinking warm coffee or broths.

Chapter 17

MY APPRECIATION

While sitting in my hospital bed recovering from the bone marrow transplant I had to wait for my blood counts to come back up and my system to be able produce enough platelets and red blood cells to sustain a healthy enough immune system. After releasing me to go home and continue with my daily Infusion Center appointments, I was sad because, I had become so used to the nursing staff that helped save my life. Throughout my illness they always helped comfort me, or put my mind at ease when I felt lost or insecure while going through my treatments.

After everything I had been through it felt like it was all coming to an end. I really learned to appreciate my life in a different way. I lived it fast and hard until I came across this disease. Being given a second chance to set better goals and take time to analyze many things that are truly more important in my life. I also met so many good and open-hearted people that are going through the ups and downs of this disease every day.

I also learned to appreciate all the doctors and nurses that continue trying to find a cure. They sacrifice so much time and effort in their own lives to save many more of the victims that did nothing wrong other than being unfortunate enough to be diagnosed with cancer. My heart goes out to all those that have lost loved ones in this struggle to overcome this disease and all other illnesses.

I also appreciate the men and women going through their own treatments on a daily basis. Most of all to all the organizations, doctors, and nurses that wake up every morning to help fight for those sick and have to witness all the suffering caused by these illnesses. Not only do they witness the suffering of the patients, but of their families as well. These people truly have hearts of gold.

What I would like to do now is thank everybody for taking the time to enjoy one of my many life experiences that I hope it can bring hope to others and their families. I know now that there are many more people out there that are experiencing or seeing someone that they love going through many dangerous treatments. These are life-saving treatments, even if the experience itself is dangerous. I would like to let you know that you are not alone in these struggles to survive.

My name is Filemon Lamas and it makes me proud to say to everyone that I am a cancer survivor and that I did not allow this disease to break me. That this disease could not stop my heart of gold! I hope that you enjoyed the journey that you just took with me and had as much fun reading it as I had living it.

Thank you for your interest and I would like to send out my best wishes and hopes to all patients and their families to stay strong throughout all you're faced with. There's always a way to smile if you take the time to look in the mirror and know that there are families and doctors fighting for you and your life. Taking this time you will then realize that you too have a heart of gold. Thank you.

Also a special thanks to the families, organizations, and facilities and their staff who participated in my recovery.